The Ultimate Mediterranean Recipes Cookbook

Don't waste the chance to make delicious and healthy lunch recipes!

Hanna Briggs

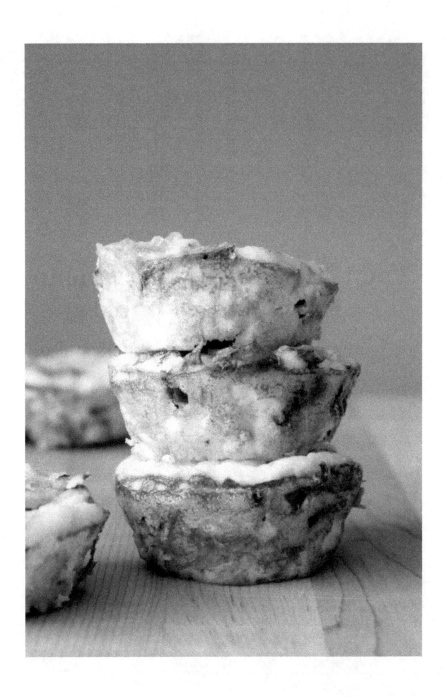

Table of contents

Introduction

Consuming the Mediterranean diet minimalizes the use of processed foods. It has been related to a reduced level of risk in developing numerous chronic diseases. It also enhances life expectancy. Several kinds of research have demonstrated many benefits in preventing cardiovascular disease, atrial fibrillation, breast cancer, and type 2 diabetes. Many pieces of evidence indicated a pattern that leads to low lipid, reduction in oxidative stress, platelet aggregation, and inflammation, and modification of growth factors and hormones involved in cancer.

Reduces Heart Diseases

According to research studies, the Mediterranean diet, which focuses on omega-3 ingredients and mono-saturated fats, reduces heart disease risk. It decreases the chances of cardiac death. The use of olive oil maintains the blood pressure levels. It is suitable for reducing hypertension. It also helps in combating the disease-promoting impacts of oxidation. This diet discourages the use of hydrogenated oils and saturated fats, which can cause heart disease.

Weight-loss

If you have been looking for diet plans for losing weight without feeling hungry, the Mediterranean diet can give you long term results. It is one of the best approaches. It is sustainable as it provides the most realistic approach to eat to feel full and energetic. This diet mostly consists of nutrient-dense food. It gives enough room for you to choose between low-carb and lower protein food. Olive oil consumed in this diet has antioxidants, natural vitamins, and some crucial fatty acids. It all improves your overall health. The Mediterranean diet focuses on natural foods, so there is very little room for junk and processed foods contributing to health-related issues and weight gain.

Most people trying the Mediterranean diet have gained positive results in cutting their weight. It is a useful option for someone looking forward to weight-loss as it provides the most unique and simple way to lose the overall calories without even changing your lifestyle that much. When you try to decrease calorie intake, losing weight is inevitable dramatically. But it will not benefit you. It will cause many health problems for you, including severe muscle loss. When you go for a Mediterranean diet, the body moves towards a sustainable model that burns calories slowly. So, it is crucial to practice the right approach and choose fat burning and more effective weight loss.

Prevents Cancer

The cornerstone of this diet is plant-based ingredients, especially vegetables and fruits. They help in preventing cancer. A plant-based diet provides antioxidants that help in protecting your DNA from damage and cell mutation. It also helps in lowering inflammation and delaying tumor growth. Various studies found that olive oil is a natural way to prevent cancer. It also decreases colon and bowel cancers. The plant-based diet balances blood sugar. It also sustains a healthy weight.

Prevents Diabetes

Numerous studies found that this healthy diet functions as an anti-inflammatory pattern, which helps fight the diseases related to chronic inflammation, Type 2 diabetes, and metabolic syndrome. It is considered very effective in preventing diabetes as it controls the insulin levels, which is a hormone to control the blood sugar levels and causes weight gain. Intake of a well-balanced diet consisting of fatty acids alongside some healthy carbohydrates and proteins is the best gift to your body. These foods help your body in burning fats more efficiently, which also provides energy. Due to the consumption of these kinds of foods, the insulin resistance level becomes non-existent, making it impossible to have high blood sugar.

Anti-aging

Choosing a Mediterranean diet without suffering from malnutrition is the most efficient and consistent anti-aging intervention. It undoubtedly expands lifespan, according to the research. The study found that the longevity biomarkers, i.e., body temperature and insulin level, and the DNA damage decreased significantly in humans by the Mediterranean diet. Other mechanisms also prove the claim made by researchers in explaining the anti-aging effects of adopting the Mediterranean diet, including reduced lipid peroxidation, high efficiency of oxidative repair, increased antioxidant defense system, and reduced mitochondrial generation rate.

Maintains Blood Sugar Level

The Mediterranean diet focuses on healthy carbs and whole grains. It has a lot of significant benefits. Consumption of whole-grain foods, like buckwheat, quinoa, and wheat berries instead of refined foods, helps you maintain blood sugar levels that ultimately gives you enough energy for the whole day.

Enhances Cognitive Health

The Mediterranean diet helps in preserving memory. It is one of the most useful steps for Alzheimer's treatment and dementia. Cognitive disorders occur when our brains do not get sufficient dopamine, which is a crucial chemical vital for mood regulation, thought processing, and body movements. Healthy fats like olive oil and nuts are good at fighting cognitive decline, mostly an age-related issue. They help counter some harmful impacts of the free radicals, inflammation, and toxins caused by having a low diet. The Mediterranean diet proves to be beneficial in decreasing

the risk of Alzheimer's to a great extent. Foods like yogurt help in having a healthy gut that improves mood, cognitive functioning, and memory.

Better Endurance Level

Mediterranean diet helps in fat loss and maintains muscle mass. It improves physical performance and enhances endurance levels. Research done on mice has shown positive results in these aspects. It also improves the health of our tissues in the long-term. The growth hormone also offers increased levels as a result of the Mediterranean diet. Which ultimately helps in improving metabolism and body composition.

Keeps You Agile

The nutrients from the Mediterranean diet reduces your risk of muscle weakness and frailty. It increases longevity. When your risk of heart disease reduces, it also reduces the risk of early death. It also strengthens your bones. Certain compounds found in olive oil help in preserving bone density. It helps increase the maturation and proliferation of the bone cells—dietary patterns of the Mediterranean diet help prevent osteoporosis.

Healthy Sleep Patterns

Our eating habits have a considerable impact on sleepiness and wakefulness. Some Mediterranean diet believers have reported an improved sleeping pattern as a result of changing their eating patterns. It has a considerable impact on your sleep because they regulate the circadian rhythm that determines our sleep patterns. If you have a regulated and balanced circadian rhythm, you will fall asleep quite quickly. You will also feel refreshed when you wake up. Another theory states that having the last meal will help you digest the food way before sleep. Digestion works best when you are upright.

Apart from focusing on plant-based eating, the Mediterranean diet philosophy emphasizes variety and moderation, living a life with perfect harmony with nature, valuing relationships in life, including sharing and enjoying meals, and having an entirely active lifestyle. The Mediterranean diet is at the crossroads. With the traditions and culture of three millennia, the Mediterranean diet lifestyle made its way to the medical world a long time ago. It has progressively recognized and became one of the successful and healthiest patterns that lead to a healthy lifestyle.

Besides metabolic, cardiovascular, cognitive, and many other benefits, this diet improves your life quality. Therefore, it is recommended today by many medical professionals worldwide. Efforts are being made in both non--Mediterranean and Mediterranean populations to make everyone benefit from the fantastic network of eating habits and patterns that began in old-time and which became a medical recommendation for a healthy lifestyle.

What to Eat and what to avoid

Fruits and vegetables: Mediterranean diet is one of the plant-based diet plans. Fresh fruits and vegetables contain a large number of vitamins, nutrients, fibers, minerals, and antioxidants

Fruits: Apple, berries, grapes, peaches, fig, grapefruit, dates, melon, oranges and pears.

Vegetables: Spinach, Brussels sprout, kale, tomatoes, kale, summer squash, onion, cauliflower, peppers, cucumbers, turnips, potatoes, sweet potatoes, and parsnips.

Seeds and nuts: Seeds and nuts are rich in monounsaturated fats and omega- 3 fatty acids.

 Seeds: pumpkin seeds, flax seeds, sesame seeds, and sunflower seeds. Nuts: Almond, hazelnuts, pistachios, cashews, and walnuts.

Whole grains: Whole grains are high in fibers and they are not processed so they do not contain unhealthy fats like trans-fats compare to processed ones.

Whole grains: Wheat, quinoa, rice, barley, oats, rye, and brown rice. You can also use bread and pasta which is made from whole grains.

Fish and seafood: Fish are the rich source of omega-3 fatty acids and proteins. Eating fish at least once a week is recommended here. The healthiest way to consume fish is to grill it. Grilling fish taste good and never need extra oil.

Fish and seafood: salmon, trout, clams, mackerel, sardines, tuna and shrimp.

Legumes: Legumes (beans) are a rich source of protein, vitamins, and fibers. Regular consumption of beans helps to reduce the risk of diabetes, cancer and heart disease.

Legumes: Kidney beans, peas, chickpeas, black beans, fava beans, lentils, and pinto beans.

Spices and herbs: Spices and herbs are used to add the taste to your meal.

Spices and herbs: mint, thyme, garlic, basil, cinnamon, nutmeg, rosemary, oregano and more.

Healthy fats: Olive oil is the main fat used in the Mediterranean diet. It helps to reduce the risk of inflammatory disorder, diabetes, cancer, and heart- related disease. It also helps to increase HDL (good cholesterol) levels and decrease LDL (bad cholesterol) levels into your body. It also helps to lose weight.

Fats: Olive oil, avocado oil, walnut oil, extra virgin olive oil, avocado, and olives.

Dairy: Moderate   amounts   of   dairy products   are   allowed   during   the Mediterranean diet. The dairy product contains high amounts of fats.

Dairy: Greek yogurt, skim milk and cheese.

Food to avoid

Refined grains: Refined grains are not allowed in a Mediterranean diet. It raises your blood sugar level. Refined grains like white bread, white rice, and pasta.

Refined oils: Oils like vegetable oils, cottonseed oils, and soybean oils are completely avoided from the Mediterranean diet. It raises your LDL (bad cholesterol) level.

Added Sugar: Added sugar is not allowed in the Mediterranean diet. These types of artificial sugars are found in table sugar, soda, chocolate, ice cream, and candies. It raises your blood sugar level.

You should consume only natural sugars in the Mediterranean diet.

Processed foods: Generally Processed foods come in boxes. Its low-fat food should not be eaten during the diet. It contains a high amount of trans-fats. Mediterranean diet is all about to eat fresh and natural food.

Trans-fat and saturated fats: In this category of food contains butter and margarine.

Processed Meat: Mediterranean diet does not allow to use of processed meat such as bacon, hot dogs and sausage.

Cabbage Curry
Servings: 4

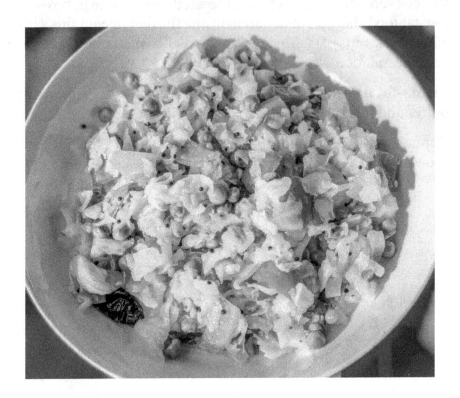

Ingredients:

- 1 head green cabbage, medium-sized
- 3 Tbs. olive oil
- ½ tsp. ground ginger
- 1 tsp. crushed dried red chilis
- ½ tsp. ground cumin
- ½ tsp. whole mustard seeds
- 2 bay leaves

- 1 tsp. ground coriander
- ½ tsp. ground turmeric
- 2 tsp. salt
- 1 cup water
- 2½ cups fresh peas
- 1 Tbs. butter
- 1½ tsp. Garam Masala
- 1 Tbs. lemon juice
- ½ tsp. sugar

Directions:

1.   Shred the cabbage coarsely. Heat the vegetable oil in a large skillet and stir in the crushed red chilis, ginger, mustard seeds, cumin, bay leaves, coriander, turmeric, and salt.

2.   Heat spices for 2 minutes whilst stirring continuously.

3.   Add the shredded cabbage and sauté it, stirring often, until it is all evenly coated with the spices and beginning to wilt, 10 to 15 minutes. Pour water over the peas. cover and cook on medium heat for 20 minutes.

4.   Remove the cover, stir in the garam masala, lemon juice, and sugar, and simmer. Serve.

Spiced Turkey w/ Avocado-Grapefruit Relish
Servings: 2

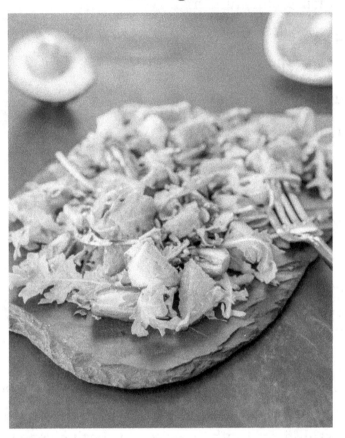

Ingredients

- Avocado-Grapefruit Relish
- 1 Large Seedless Grapefruit
- 1 Small Minced Shallot
- 1 teaspoon of Red Wine Vinegar
- 1/2 Small Avocado (Pitted, Peeled, & Diced)
- 1 teaspoon of Honey
- tablespoon of Chopped Fresh Cilantro Spiced Turkey

- 8-ounce Turkey Cutlets

- 1/2 teaspoon of Five-Spice Powder

- 1 tablespoon of Chili Powder

- 1 tablespoon of Canola Oil

- 1/8 teaspoon of Salt

Directions:

1. Remove peel and the white pith from your grapefruit using a sharp knife. Discard it. Cut your grapefruit into segments from the surrounding membrane, allowing them to drop into your small-sized bowl. Squeeze out the juice that remains into your bowl and discard the membrane. Add your shallots, vinegar, cilantro, honey, and avocado. Toss it well to combine. Set to the side.

2. Combine your five-spice powder, chili powder, and salt on a plate. Put your turkey into the spice mixture and coat well.

3. Heat your oil over a medium-high heat in a medium-sized skillet. Add your turkey and cook for 2 to 3 minutes per side until there is no pink left in the middle. Remove from heat.

4. Divide turkey onto 2 separate plates. Add your avocado-grapefruit relish on the side.

5. Serve and Enjoy!

Oriental-Style Chicken Noodle Soup
Servings: 4

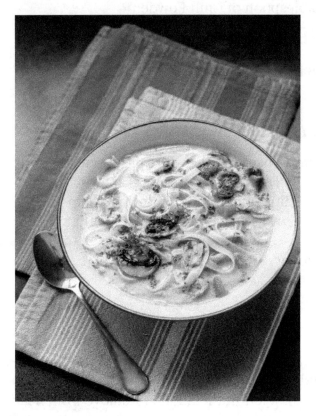

Ingredients:

- 12 oz skinless chicken breasts, cut into thin strips
- 4 cups napa cabbage, chopped
- pack rice noodles
- 6 scallions, sliced thinly on the bias
- 8 cups chicken broth
- 4 tablespoons rice vinegar
- ½ cup cilantro leaves, chopped clove garlic, minced

- ½ teaspoon Vietnamese chile paste

- 4 tablespoons soy sauce

- 2 tablespoons ginger, minced

- 2 tablespoons mirin tablespoon sugar

- 1 teaspoon dark sesame oil

Directions:

1.   In a small bowl, combine mirin, 1 teaspoon sesame oil, soy sauce, sugar, vinegar, chile paste, garlic and ginger. Set aside.

2.   In a medium saucepan, heat broth over medium heat. Stir in soy sauce mixture and chicken. Add all vegetables and bring to a boil. Reduce heat and simmer for 2 minutes or until chicken is fully cooked. Add another teaspoon of sesame oil. Stir and season as you wish.

3.   Meanwhile, cook rice noodles according to package directions. Drain and transfer in serving bowl.

4.   Pour hot soup over prepared noodles. Top with scallions and cilantro. Serve hot.

Tortellini with Broccoli and Pesto
Servings: 2

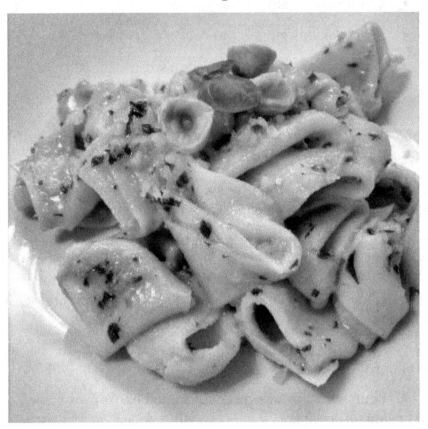

Ingredients:

- 8 cherry tomatoes, halved

- 3 tablespoons pesto (fresh, if possible)

- 250 g fresh tortellini

- 2 tablespoons toasted pine nut

- 140 g tender stem broccoli, cut into short lengths

- tablespoon balsamic vinegar

Directions:

1.   Pour water into a large pan; bring to a boil.

2.   When the water is boiling, add the broccoli; cook for 2 minutes. Add the tortellini; cook for 2 minutes. Or, cook the vegetables according to the package directions. When cooked, drain and cool under running water. Transfer into a large mixing bowl.

3.   Add the pesto, the pine nuts, and the vinegar; toss to combine.

4.   Add the tomatoes; divide between two containers, then chill in the fridge.

5.   When ready to serve, allow to thaw to room temperature.

Tuna Sandwiches
Servings: 4

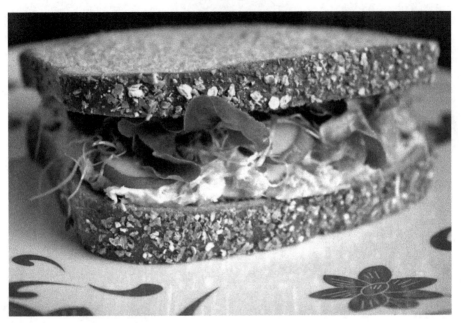

Ingredients:

- 1/3 cup sun-dried tomato packed in oil, drained

- 1/4 cup red bell pepper, finely chopped (optional)

- 1/4 cup red onions or 1⁄4 cup sweet Spanish onion, finely chopped

- 1/4 cup ripe green olives or 1⁄4 cup ripe olives, sliced

- 1/4 teaspoon black pepper, fresh ground

- 2 cans (6 ounce) tuna in water, drained, flaked

- 2 teaspoons capers (more to taste)

- 4 romaine lettuce or curly green lettuce leaves

- 4 teaspoons balsamic vinegar

- 4 teaspoons roasted red pepper
- 8 slices whole-grain bread (or 8 slices whole-wheat pita bread)
- Olive oil

Optional:

- 3 tablespoons mayonnaise (or low-fat mayonnaise)

Directions:

1.   Toast the bread, if desired.

2.   In a small mixing bowl, mix the vinegar and the olive oil. Brush the oil mixture over 1 side of each bread slices or on the inside of the pita pockets.

3.   Except for the lettuce, combine the remaining of the ingredients in a mixing bowl.

4.   Place 1 lettuce leaf on the oiled side of 4 bread slices.

5.   Top the leaves with the tuna mix; top with the remaining bread slices with the oiled side in.

6.   If using pita, place 1 lettuce leave inside each pita slices, then fill with the tuna mixture; serve immediately

Roasted Summer Vegetables Layers
Servings: 4

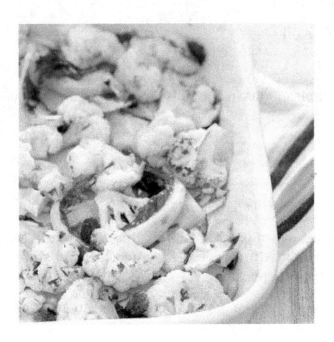

Ingredients:

- Large garlic bulb, kept whole
- Small bunch rosemary, broken into sprigs
- Aubergines/eggplants, sliced
- Large courgettes/zucchini, sliced into thick pieces (yellow ones preferred)
- ripe plum tomato, sliced tablespoons olive oil, good quality

Directions:

1. Preheat the oven to 220C, gas to 7, or fan to 200C.

2. Grease a round oven-safe dish with a little olive oil

3.   Starting from the outside, alternately layer the vegetable slices, making a concentric circle until you fill the dish to the middle. Place the whole garlic in the center of the layer. If there are any leftover vegetable slices, tuck them into gaps in the layer, around the outside. Stick rosemary sprigs between the vegetables and then generously drizzle with olive oil; season with salt and pepper.

4.   Roast for about 50 minutes up to 1 hour, or until the layered vegetables are lightly charred and soft.

5.   Remove the dish from the dish; let stand for a couple of minutes.

6.   Remove the whole garlic head, separate the cloves, and serve for squeezing over the vegetables.

Sumac Salmon and Grapefruit
Servings: 4

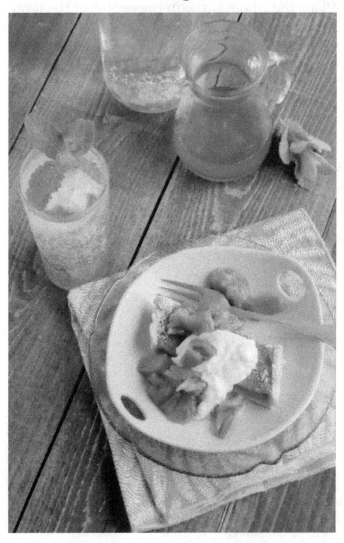

Ingredients:

- Cup parsley leaves, flat-leaf
- Teaspoon ground cumin

- 1/4 cup (60ml) olive oil, plus more to brush Oranges, peeled, segmented
- Pink grapefruits, peeled, segmented
- 2 Tablespoons sumac
- Pieces (180 g each) salmon fillets, skinless, pin-boned
- Juice of 1/2 lemon, and wedges to serve

Directions:

1.	In a mixing bowl, combine the sumac and the cumin.

2.	Brush the fillets with the olive oil; season with the sumac mixture.

3.	In a large frying pan, heat 1 tablespoon olive oil over medium heat. Add the fish fillets; cook for about 2 minutes per side, or until charred on the outside and almost cooked through, but still pink in the middle. Transfer to a plate and loosely cover with foil.

4.	Meanwhile, whisk the remaining 2 tablespoons of olive oil and lemon juice; season. Add the fruits and the parsley, toss to coat.

5.	Serve the fish fillets with the salad and wedges of lemon.

Mediterranean Bow
Servings: 6

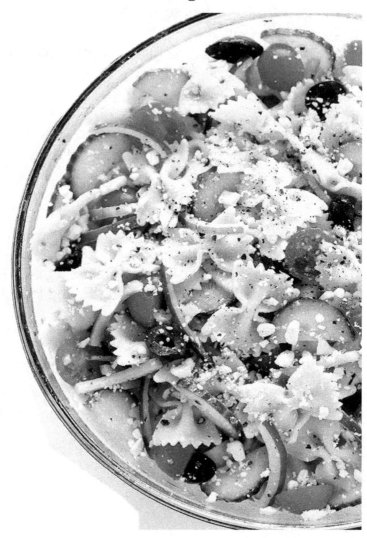

Ingredients:

- Small red onion, thinly sliced
- 1 yellow bell pepper, deseeded, thinly sliced

- 1/2 cup basil leaves, torn
- 185 g green olives stuffed with feta, halved
- Large tomatoes, vine-ripened, chopped
- 2 Tablespoons baby capers, drained
- 300 g bowtie pasta
- Slices prosciutto

For the dressing:

- 1 garlic clove, crushed
- 1 tablespoon balsamic vinegar
- 1 teaspoon caster sugar
- 1 teaspoon dried chili flakes
- 1/4 cup olive oil
- 1/4 cup red wine vinegar or sweet sherry
- 2 teaspoons dijon mustard

Directions:

1.   Over high heat, heat a nonstick frying pan. When the pan is hot, add the prosciutto; cook for 3 minutes per side or until crispy. Set aside and let cool

2.   Meanwhile, cook the pasta in a large saucepan with salted boiling water according to the package directions until tender. Drain and then rinse under warm running water. Transfer into a large-sized bowl.

3.   Add the bell peppers, tomato, onion, olive, capers, and basil into the pasta. Crumble the crispy prosciutto over. Gently toss to combine.

4.   Whisk all of the dressing ingredients together until well mixed.

5.   Drizzle the dressing over the salad, season the salt and pepper, and gently toss; serve.

Greek Crispy Pie
Servings: 4

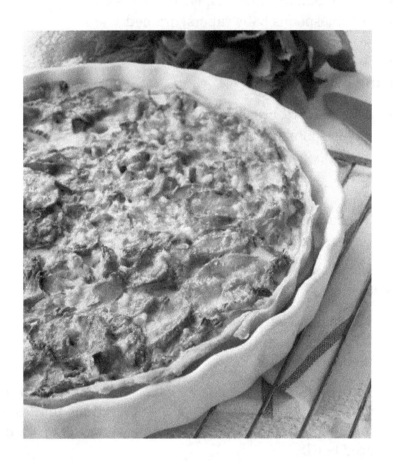

Ingredients:

- 1/2 of a 250 g pack whole-wheat filo pastry
- 200 g bag spinach
- 2 eggs
- 100 g feta cheese, crumbled
- 175 g jar sundried tomato in oil, reserve oil

Directions:

1.   Place the spinach in a large skillet or pan. Pour a couple of tablespoons water; cook until just wilted. Drain into a colander or sieve. Let cool, squeeze to remove excess water, and then roughly chop; put into a mixing bowl.

2.   Roughly chop tomatoes and add into the bowl with spinach. Crack the eggs into the bowl and then add the feta; mix well.

3.   Carefully unroll the pastry. Cover with damped pieces of paper towel to prevent it from drying. Take 1 sheet of pastry, liberally brush 1 side of it with some of the reserved tomato oil.

4.   With the oiled side down, place the pastry into a loose-bottomed 22 cm cake tin. Some parts of the pastry will hang over the cake tin sides.

5.   Brush another pastry with the tomato oil and then place in the cake tin a little further from the first one. Layer another oiled pastry until you have three layers.

6.   Pour the filling. Pull over the pastry sides towards the middle to cover the filling. Scrunch up the pastry, making sure the filling is fully covered and then brush with more tomato oil.

7.   Heat an oven to 180C, gas to 4, or fan to 160C.

8.   Cook the pie for about 30 minutes, or until the pastry is golden and crisp.

9.   Remove from the tin and slice into 4 wedges; serve with Mediterranean salad.

Mediterranean Pasta with Basil
Servings: 4

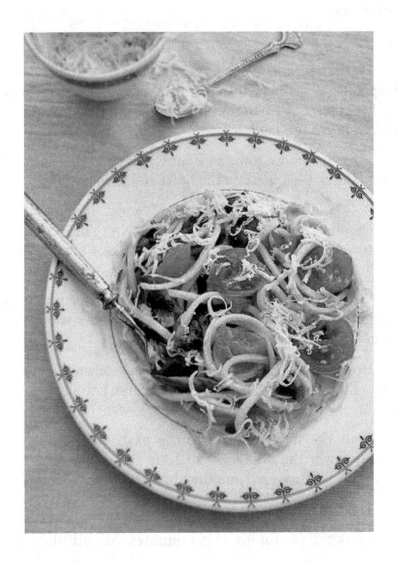

Ingredients:

- 350 g dried pasta (whole-wheat corkscrew)
- 3 garlic cloves, coarsely chopped
- 2 tablespoons olive oil, plus more to serve
- 2 red peppers, seeded, cut into chunks
- 2 red onions, cut into wedges

- 2 mild red chili, seeded, diced teaspoon golden caster sugar
- 1 kg small ripe tomatoes, quartered tablespoon
- grated Parmesan, to serve
- 1 handful fresh basil leaves, to serve

Directions:

1.   To roast the vegetables:

2.   Preheat gas oven to 200C, gas to 6, or fan to 180C.

3.   Scatter the peppers, the red peppers, the chilies, and the garlic into a large-sized roasting tin.

4.   Sprinkle with the sugar and then drizzle with the olive oil; season well with the salt and the pepper.

5.   Roast for about 15 minutes. Toss the tomatoes in the tin and then roast for additional 15 minutes, or until the vegetables are soft and golden.

6.   For the pasta:

7.   While the vegetables are roasting, cook the pasta according to the instructions of the package until tender with still a little bit of bite; drain well.

8.   Remove the roasted vegetables from oven. Add the pasta into the tin; toss lightly to mix.

9.   Tear the basil leaves and sprinkle over the pasta mixture. Sprinkle with the parmesan cheese.

Homemade Self-Rising Whole-Wheat Flour
Servings: 1

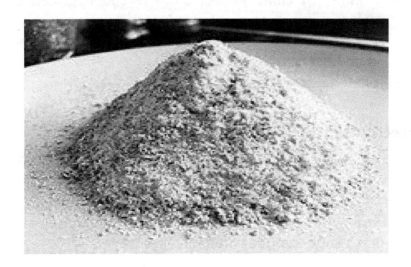

Ingredients:

- Cup (140 grams or 4 7/8 ounces) whole-wheat flour
- 1⁄4-1⁄2 teaspoon salt
- 1 1⁄4 teaspoons baking powder

Directions:

1. Combine all of the ingredients in a large-sized airtight container; shake well to combine, and then cover.

Creamy Mediterranean Paninis
Servings: 4

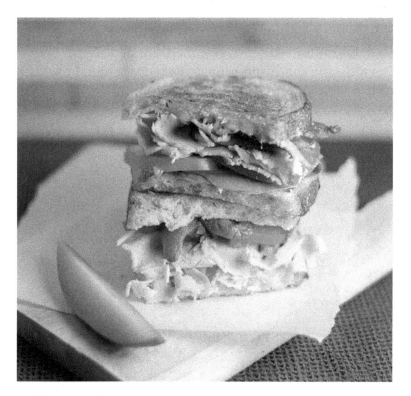

Ingredients:

- 1/2 cup of Mayonnaise w/ Olive Oil (divided)

- 1/4 cup of Chopped Fresh Basil Leaves

- 1 Small Thinly Sliced Zucchini

- 2 tablespoons of Finely Chopped Black Olives

- 4 slices of Provolone Cheese

- 7 ounces of Sliced Roasted Red Peppers

- 8 slices of 1/2 Inch Thick Whole Grain Bread

Directions:

1.   Combine your mayonnaise w/ olive oil, basil, and black olives in a bowl. Evenly spread your bread slices with this mixture. Layer 4 slices of bread with zucchini, peppers, bacon, and provolone. Top with your remaining 4 slices of bread.

2.   Spread some mayonnaise on outside of your sandwiches and cook them in a skillet over a medium heat. Turn them once, cooking until the sandwiches have turned a golden brown and the cheese has melted. Should take about 4 minutes.

Fresh Tomato Pasta Bowl
Servings: 4

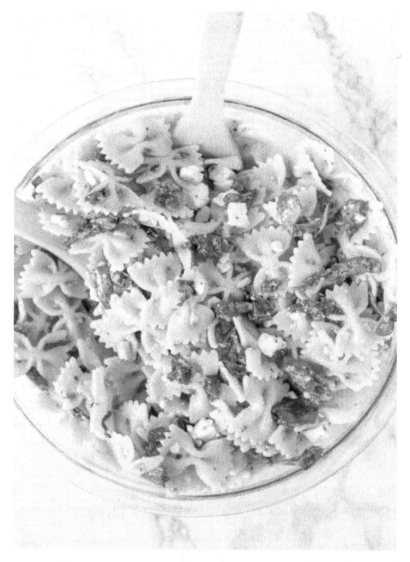

Ingredients

- 8 ounces whole-grain linguine
- 1 tablespoon extra-virgin olive oil

- 2 garlic cloves, minced

- 1/4 cup chopped yellow onion

- 1 teaspoon chopped fresh oregano

- 1/2 teaspoon salt

- 1/4 teaspoon freshly ground black pepper

- 1 teaspoon tomato paste

- 8 ounces cherry tomatoes, halved

- 1/2 cup grated Parmesan cheese

- 1 tablespoon chopped fresh parsley

Directions

1.	Bring a large saucepan of water to a boil over high heat and cook the linguine according to the package instructions until al dente (still slightly firm). Drain, reserving 1/2 cup of the pasta water. Do not rinse the pasta.

2.	In a large, heavy skillet, heat the olive oil over medium-high heat. Sauté the garlic, onion, and oregano until the onion is just translucent, about 5 minutes.

3.	Add the salt, pepper, tomato paste, and 1/4 cup of the reserved pasta water. Stir well and allow it to cook for 1 minute.

4.	Stir in the tomatoes and cooked pasta, tossing everything well to coat. Add more pasta water if needed.

5.	To serve, mound the pasta in shallow bowls and top with Parmesan cheese and parsley.

Cheesy Stuffed Tomatoes
Servings: 2

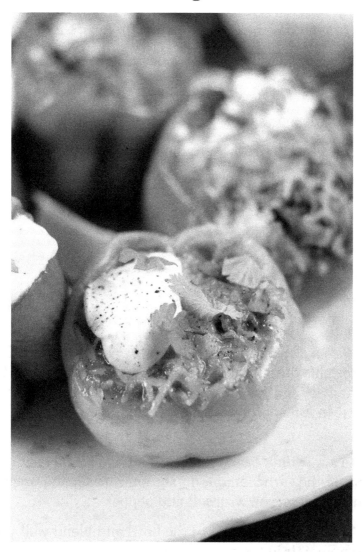

Ingredients

- 4 large, ripe tomatoes
- 1 tablespoon extra-virgin olive oil

- 2 garlic cloves, minced

- 1/2 cup diced yellow onion

- 1/2 pound white or cremini mushrooms, sliced

- 1 tablespoon chopped fresh basil

- 1 tablespoon chopped fresh oregano

- 1/2 teaspoon salt

- 1/4 teaspoon freshly ground black pepper

- 1 cup shredded part-skim mozzarella cheese

- 1 tablespoon grated Parmesan cheese

Directions

1.   Preheat the oven to 375°F. Line a baking sheet with aluminum foil.

2.   Slice a sliver from the bottom of each tomato so they will stand upright without wobbling. Cut a 1/2-inch slice from the top of each tomato and use a spoon to gently remove most of the pulp, placing it in a medium bowl. Place the tomatoes on the baking sheet.

3.   In a medium, heavy skillet, heat the olive oil over medium heat. Sauté the garlic, onion, mushrooms, basil, and oregano for 5 minutes, and season with salt and pepper.

4.   Transfer the mixture to the bowl and blend well with the tomato pulp. Stir in the mozzarella cheese.

5.   Fill each tomato loosely with the mixture, top with Parmesan cheese, and bake until the cheese is bubbly, 15 to 20 minutes. Serve immediately.

Tortellini with Broccoli and Pesto
Servings: 2

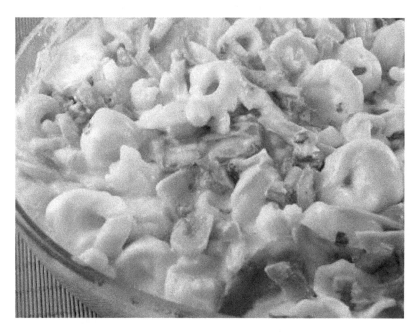

Ingredients:

- 8 cherry tomatoes, halved
- 3 tablespoons pesto (fresh, if possible)
- 250 g fresh tortellini
- 2 tablespoons toasted pine nut
- 140 g tender stem broccoli, cut into short lengths
  Tablespoon balsamic vinegar

Directions:

1. Pour water into a large pan; bring to a boil.

2. When the water is boiling, add the broccoli; cook for 2 minutes. Add the tortellini; cook for 2 minutes. Or, cook the vegetables according to the package directions. When cooked, drain and cool under running water. Transfer into a large mixing bowl.

3. Add the pesto, the pine nuts, and the vinegar; toss to combine.

4. Add the tomatoes; divide between two containers, then chill in the fridge.

5. When ready to serve, allow to thaw to room temperature.

Tuna Sandwiches
Servings: 4

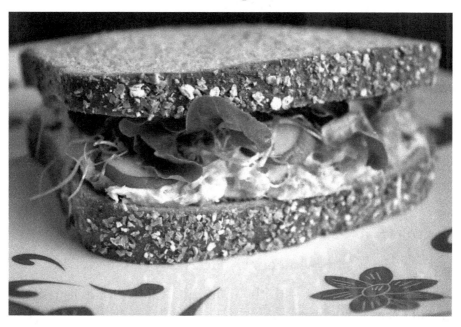

Ingredients:

- 1/3 cup sun-dried tomato packed in oil, drained
- 1/4 cup red bell pepper, finely chopped (optional)
- 1/4 cup red onions or 1⁄4 cup sweet Spanish onion, finely chopped
- 1/4 cup ripe green olives or 1⁄4 cup ripe olives, sliced
- 1/4 teaspoon black pepper, fresh ground
- 2 cans (6 ounce) tuna in water, drained, flaked
- 2 teaspoons capers (more to taste)
- 4 romaine lettuce or curly green lettuce leaves
- 4 teaspoons balsamic vinegar
- 4 teaspoons roasted red pepper
- 8 slices whole-grain bread (or 8 slices whole-wheat pita bread) Olive oil

Optional:

- 3 tablespoons mayonnaise (or low-fat mayonnaise)

Directions:

1.   Toast the bread, if desired.

2.   In a small mixing bowl, mix the vinegar and the olive oil. Brush the oil mixture over 1 side of each bread slices or on the inside of the pita pockets.

3.   Except for the lettuce, combine the remaining of the ingredients in a mixing bowl.

4.   Place 1 lettuce leaf on the oiled side of 4 bread slices.

5.   Top the leaves with the tuna mix; top with the remaining bread slices with the oiled side in.

6.   If using pita, place 1 lettuce leave inside each pita slices, then fill with the tuna mixture; serve immediately.

Mediterranean Scallops
Servings: 4

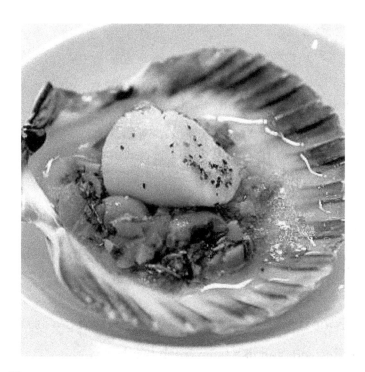

Ingredients:

- 8 to 12 ounces whole-wheat linguine
- 2 teaspoons garlic, minced
- 2 tablespoons shallots, minced
- 1/4 teaspoon salt substitute
- 1/4 teaspoon black pepper, freshly ground
- Tablespoon olive oil
- 1 tablespoon dried basil, crushed
- 1 pinch red pepper flakes, crushed
- 1 pound sea scallops, cut crosswise into halves 1 can (8 ounces) tomato sauce, no-salt-added

- 1 can (14 1/2 ounces) whole tomatoes, no-salt-added, drain, chop, reserve juice

Directions:

1.   In a large skillet or pan on medium heat. Add the garlic and the shallots; sauté for about 1 minute.

2.   Add the chopped tomatoes with the juice, the tomato sauce, the herbs, and season with the salt and the pepper; stir and simmer for 10 minutes.

3.   Add the scallops; continue cooking gently for 5 minutes, or until the scallops are just cooked through.

4.   Meanwhile, cook the linguine according to the direction of the package until al dente; drain and divide between 4 pasta bowls, about 1 cup for each bowl.

5.   Divide the scallop mixture between the 4 bowls.

6.   If desired, garnish with fresh basil leaves.

7.   Serve with whole-grain Italian bread and tosses green salad.

8.   Serve immediately.

Mediterranean-Style Salmon Fillet
Servings: 6

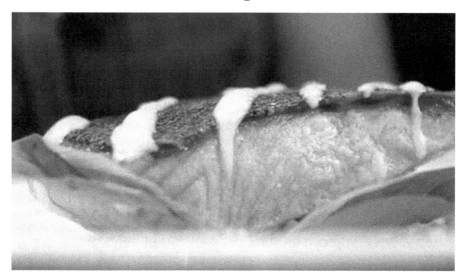

Ingredients:

- whole (about 800 g or 28.2 oz.) salmon fillet, skin-on, well- trimmed (organic is preferred)
- 18 pieces black olives (preferably Niçoise), pitted
- 9 marinated sundried tomato, halved
- tablespoons olive oil 18 pieces basil leaves

Directions:

1.   Preheat the oven to 200C, gas to 6, or fan to 180C.

2.   Place the salmon fillet on a clean cutting board. With an apple corer, create 3 rows of 6 holes in the length of the fillet, making 18 holes in all and going just down until it reaches the skin, but not holing all the way through.

3.   With a basil leaf, wrap together 1 piece of sundried tomato and 1 piece of olive together, rolling the leaf to make a tight parcel that is big enough to fit the holes.

4.   Stuff the parcels into each holes in the fillet.

5.   Put the salmon into foiled and then greased baking tray; season with salt, pepper, and then drizzle with the 3 tablespoons olive oil.

6.   Place the tray in the oven; roast for about 20 minutes or until the salmon is just cooked.

7.   Remove the tray from the oven, let cool until the fillet is just warm. Carefully transfer the fillet onto a serving dish; serve.

Alternatively, you can let the fillet cool completely.

Roasted Summer Vegetables Layers
Servings: 4

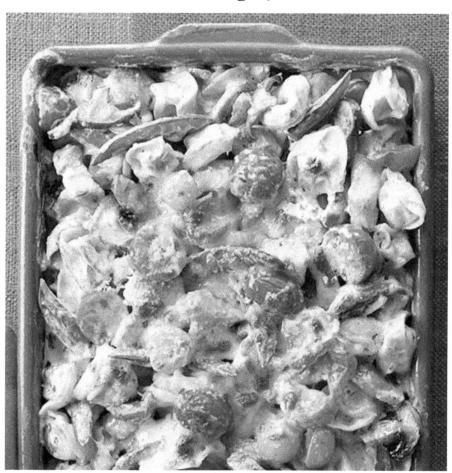

Ingredients:

- Large garlic bulb, kept whole
- Small bunch rosemary, broken into sprigs
- Aubergines/eggplants, sliced
- Large courgettes/zucchini, sliced into thick pieces (yellow ones preferred)
- Ripe plum tomato, sliced

- Tablespoons olive oil, good-quality

Directions:

1.   Preheat the oven to 220C, gas to 7, or fan to 200C.

2.   Grease a round oven-safe dish with a little olive oil

3.   Starting from the outside, alternately layer the vegetable slices, making a concentric circle until you fill the dish to the middle. Place the whole garlic in the center of the layer. If there are any leftover vegetable slices, tuck them into gaps in the layer, around the outside. Stick rosemary sprigs between the vegetables and then generously drizzle with olive oil; season with salt and pepper.

4.   Roast for about 50 minutes up to 1 hour, or until the layered vegetables are lightly charred and soft.

5.   Remove the dish from the dish; let stand for a couple of minutes.

6.   Remove the whole garlic head, separate the cloves, and serve for squeezing over the vegetables.

Mediterranean Halibut Sandwiches
Servings: 4

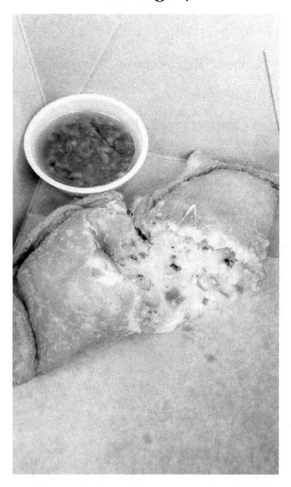

Ingredients: Fish:

- Vegetable Oil Cooking Spray

- 12 ounce Center Cut Skinned Halibut Fillet

- 1/4 teaspoon of Freshly Ground Black Pepper

- 1/2 teaspoon of Kosher Salt

- Extra-Virgin Olive Oil Bread:
- 1 loaf of Ciabatta Bread
- 1 clove of Peeled Garlic
- 2 tablespoons of Extra-Virgin Olive Oil Filling:
- 1/3 cup of Mayonnaise
- 1/4 cup of Chopped Fresh Basil Leaves
- 1/4 cup of Chopped Sun-Dried Tomatoes
- 1 tablespoon of Drained Capers
- Zest of 1 Large Lemon
- 2 cups of Arugula
- 1/4 teaspoon of Ground Black Pepper
- 1/2 teaspoon of Kosher Salt

Directions:

For your fish

1. Place your oven rack in the middle of your oven. Preheat your oven to 450 degrees. Spray your baking dish with vegetable oil cooking spray. Set to the side.

2. Season your halibut on both sides with your pepper and salt. Place on your baking sheet. Drizzle with olive oil. Bake until your fish is cooked all the way through and the skins flakes easily with a fork. Should take approximately 10 to 15 minutes. Set to the side for 20 minutes to cool.

For your bread

1.   Preheat a skillet over a medium-high heat. Remove a little of the dough from the top half of the bread. Make sure the ends of the bread are trimmed off and the bread is halved.

2.   Brush the cut sides of your bread with olive oil.

3.   Grill the bread until it is golden. Should take 1 to 2 minutes.

4.   Rub the cooked surface with the cut side of your garlic. For your filling

1.   Combine the mayonnaise, basil, sun-dried tomatoes, capers, parsley, salt, lemon zest, and pepper in a bowl.

2.   Using your fork, flake the fish you set to the side and add your filling. Mix until it is all incorporated. Place your filling on the bottom half of your bread. Top it with arugula. Add the top half of your bread and cut it into four sandwiches of equal size.

3.   Serve and Enjoy!

Mediterranean Chickpea Patties
Servings: 4

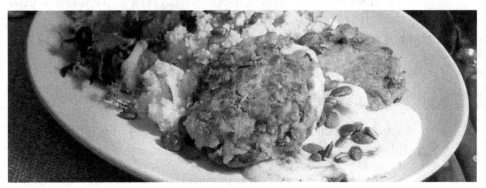

Ingredients:

- 15-ounce can of Chickpeas
- 1 clove of Chopped Garlic
- 1/2 cup of Fresh Parsley
- 1/4 teaspoon of Ground Cumin
- 1/2 teaspoon of Black Pepper
- 1/2 teaspoon of Kosher Salt
- 1 Egg
- 2 tablespoons of Olive Oil
- 4 tablespoons of Flour
- 3 tablespoons of Fresh Lemon Juice
- 1/2 cup of Low-Fat Greek Style Yogurt
- 8 cups of Mixed Salad Greens
- 1/2 Small Thinly Sliced Red Onion
- 1 cup of Grape Tomatoes

- Pita Chips

Directions:

1.   Pulse your chickpeas, garlic, parsley, cumin, pepper, and salt in a food processor until everything is chopped coarsely and your mixture comes together. Transfer over to a bowl, add your egg and 2 tablespoons of flour. Form into 8 patties each 1/2 inch thick in size. Place your remaining flour in a dish and roll your patties in it. Tap off your excess flour.

2.   Heat oil in a skillet over a medium-high heat. Cook your patties for 2 to 3 minutes per side until golden.

3.   Whisk together your yogurt, lemon juice, and a dash of salt and pepper. Divide your greens, onion, tomatoes, and patties evenly among your 4 plates. Drizzle each of your salads with 2 tablespoons of dressing. Add pita chips on the side.

4.   Serve and Enjoy!

Chicken w/ Mustard Greens, Olives, and Lemon
Servings: 6

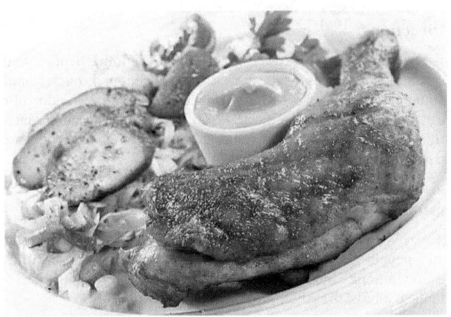

Ingredients:

- 6 Bone-In Skinless Chicken Breast Halves

- 2 tablespoons of Olive Oil

- 1 Medium Thinly Sliced Red Onion

- 4 cloves of Mashed Garlic

- 1 1/2 pounds of Mustard Greens w/ Stalks Removed

- 1 cup of Dry White Wine

- 1/2 cup of Pitted Kalamata Olive

- 1 tablespoon of Lemon Juice

- Coarse Salt

- Ground Pepper

- Lemon Wedges (Optional)

Directions:

1.   In a 5-quart Dutch oven, heat 1 tablespoon of oil over a medium-high heat. Season your chicken with pepper and salt.

Add half of your chicken to your Dutch oven and cook it until it is browned on every side. Should take approximately 6 to 8 minutes. Transfer to your plate. Repeat with the remaining oil and the remaining chicken.

2.   Add your garlic and onion to an oven. Cook for 4 to 6 minutes until softened. Add your wine and chicken (along with any juices) to the skillet and bring it to a boil. Reduce your heat to a medium heat and cook approximately 5 minutes.

3.   Place your greens on top of your chicken. Season with your pepper and salt. Cover and continue to cook chicken until it's opaque throughout and all your greens have wilted. Should take around 3 to 5 minutes.

4.   Remove it from the heat and stir in your olives and lemon juice.

5.   Transfer to a plate and drizzle the chicken juice over top your chicken. Can add optional lemon wedges on the side if you so desire.

6.   Serve and Enjoy!

Vegetable Curry
Servings: 4

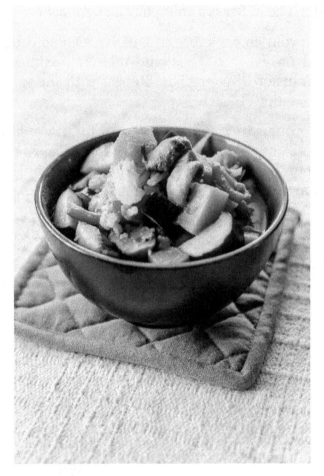

Ingredients:

- ¼ cup olive oil
- 3 cloves garlic, minced
- Tbs. peeled and grated fresh ginger
- ½ cup chopped onions
- 1 tsp. mustard seeds
- Tbs. ground coriander

- 1 tsp. ground turmeric
- ¼ tsp. cayenne pepper 1 cup thin-sliced carrots
- ½ lb. string beans, cut in 1-inch lengths
- 1 cup sliced green onions
- Green bell peppers, stemmed, seeded, and cut in strips
- 1 small, hot green chili, minced
- cup flaked unsweetened coconut 2 cups water
- 1½ tsp. salt
- tsp. sugar
- ½ cup peeled, sliced pimiento pepper
- ⅔ cup yogurt

Directions:

1.   Heat the oil in a large, heavy-bottomed skillet and sauté the garlic, ginger, and onions in it until the onions begin to show color.

2.   Add the mustard seeds, coriander, turmeric, and cayenne, and stir over medium heat for about 2 minutes.

3.   Add the carrots, string beans, green onions, bell peppers, and hot chili and toss with the spices for a few minutes, then add the coconut, water, salt, and sugar. Stir well. Allow to simmer for 20 minutes.

4.   Remove the lid and continue simmering, stirring often, until the liquid is reduced by over half.

5.   Stir in the pimiento strips and yogurt, cook a few minutes more over high heat, and taste. Correct the seasoning if necessary and serve hot with rice and raitas.

Penne Mushrooms and Squash
Servings: 4

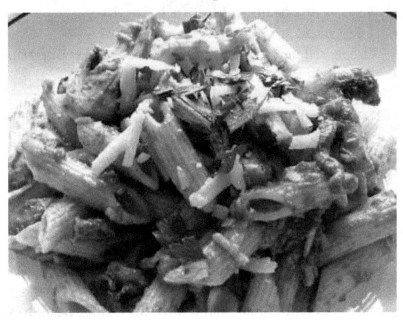

Ingredients:

- 2 cups butternut squash
- 12 ounces penne pasta
- 2 tablespoons olive oil (extra-virgin)
- freshly ground pepper (to taste)
- 1/4 teaspoon red pepper flakes
- 4 cloves garlic
- 12 ounces mushrooms kosher salt (to taste)
- cup grated parmesan cheese
- 1/2 small red onion tablespoons fresh oregano

Directions:

1. In a large skillet, pour salted water and bring to a rolling boil; add pasta.

2. Once the penne is al dente, reserve a cup of pasta water and drain the rest.

3. Meanwhile, prepare a large skillet, add the squash, pepper and salt; cook until tender.

4. In the same skillet, add the mushrooms. Olive oil, pepper and salt then cook for 5 minutes.

5. Toss in the red pepper flakes and shallot; stir until tender.

6. When the pasta is done, add the penne, penne water and squash, heat the skillet through.

7. Transfer on a large plate; garnish with oregano and parmesan cheese.

Corned Beef and Cabbage
Servings: 6

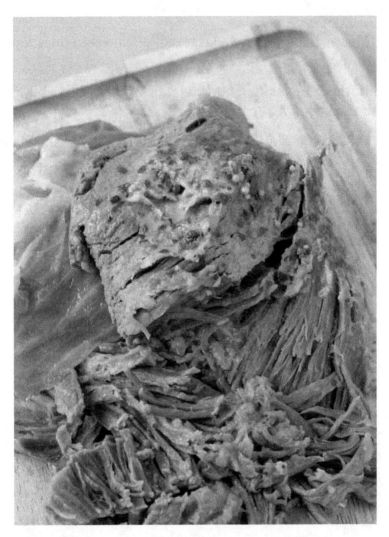

Ingredients:

- 2lbs corned beef brisket with seasoning pack
- 4 medium carrots, cut into 1-inch cubes
- 4 medium unpeeled red potatoes, cut into 1-inch cubes
- large cabbage, cut into 8 wedges

- 1 12oz can beer
- 1 medium onion, wedged
- Water
- Sauce
- 1 tsp dijon mustard
- ¼ apple sauce

Directions:

1.   Apply cooking spray to a 6-quart slow cooker. Put carrots, potatoes and onions.

2.   Place corned beef brisket on top and sprinkle with contents of seasoning pack. Add beer and water, just right above the beef brisket.

3.   Cook on low for 10 to 12 hours. Remove beef from cooker, place on a platter and keep warm.

4.   Meanwhile, throw in the cabbage in the slow cooker and set temperature to high. Cover and cook for 30 minutes or until cabbage is crispy and tender. Skim excess fat from broth.

5.   In a small bowl, combine apple sauce and Dijon mustard.

6.   Cut cooked corned beef brisket into thin slices. Place cooked vegetables on a platter and arrange corned beef slices on top. Add some broth left in the cooker. Sprinkle with sauce mixture.

Asparagus and Salmon in a Foil
Servings: 4

Ingredients:

- 5 ounces salmon fillets
- Lemon, fresh
- 1 lb. asparagus
- Black pepper, freshly ground Lemon wedges, for garnish
- Salt

Directions:

1.   Preheat oven to about 450 degrees F.

2.   Remove the ends off asparagus spears (snapping them off at the tender part will do the trick) and then separate into 4 portions.

3.   Spray non-stick cooking spray on the center of each foil sheet. Place one fillet at the center of each sheet, and then top with one portion of the asparagus. Squeeze lemon juice onto the stalks.

4.   Add ground pepper and salt or any seasoning blend.

5.   Pull up the sides of the wrap and then fold the top over two times.

6.   Seal the edges but leave enough room in the wrapped packets for air to circulate.

7.   Place the packets on a cookie sheet. Place in oven until salmon looks opaque (which should take about 15 to 18 minutes). Reminder: Please be careful when opening the foil packets because the steam is very hot.

8. Garnish with lemon wedges. Serve.

Two-Cheeses Baked Potato
Servings: 5

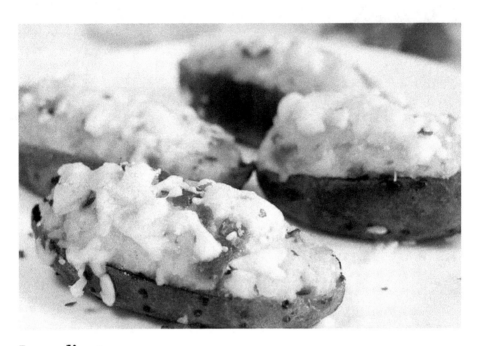

Ingredients:

- 4 baking potatoes, large,
- baked 2 cups cheddar cheese, shredded
- tablespoon parmesan cheese, grated
- tablespoons olive oil
- 1/4 teaspoon garlic powder
- 1/4 teaspoon paprika
- 1/2 teaspoon salt
- 1/8 teaspoon pepper

Directions:

1.   Cut potatoes into halves, lengthwise. Scoop the pulp out (to save or to use later for another recipe – your choice) to leave 1/4-inch shells.

2.   Place potatoes on a greased baking sheet.

3.   Combine Parmesan, oil, salt, paprika, garlic powder, and pepper and then brush mixture all over the potato skins.

4.   Bake at a temperature of 475°F for around 8 minutes before turning over. Bake for 8 more minutes before turning them right side up.

5.   Evenly sprinkle cheddar inside the skins.

6.   Bake for 2 minutes more or until parmesan melts.

Garlicky Broiled Sardines
Servings: 4

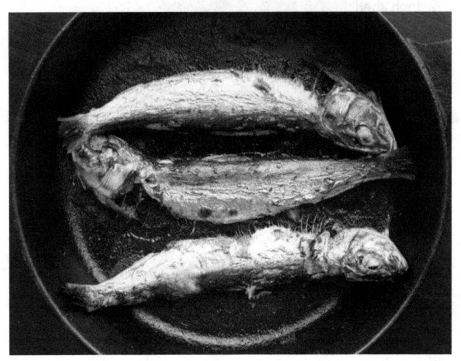

Ingredients

- 4 (3.25-ounce) cans sardines (about 16 sardines), packed in water or olive oil

- 2 tablespoons extra-virgin olive oil (if sardines are packed in water)

- • 4 garlic cloves, minced

- 1/2 teaspoon red pepper flakes

- 1/2 teaspoon salt

- • 1/4 teaspoon freshly ground black pepper

Directions

1.   Preheat the broiler. Line a baking dish with aluminum foil. Arrange the sardines in a single layer on the foil.

2.   Combine the olive oil (if using), garlic, and red pepper flakes in a small bowl and spoon over each sardine. Season with salt and pepper.

3.   Broil just until sizzling, 2 to 3 minutes.

4.   To serve, place 4 sardines on each plate and top with any remaining garlic mixture that has collected in the baking dish.

Fruited Chicken Salad
Servings: 2

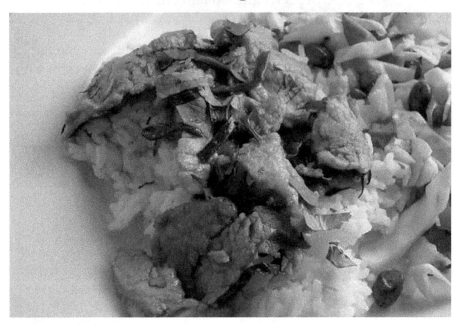

Ingredients

- 2 cups chopped cooked chicken breast
- 2 Granny Smith apples, peeled, cored, and diced
- 1/2 cup dried cranberries
- 1/4 cup diced red onion
- 1/4 cup diced celery
- 2 tablespoons honey Dijon mustard
- 1 tablespoon olive oil mayonnaise
- 1/2 teaspoon salt
- 1/4 teaspoon freshly ground black pepper

Directions

1.	In a medium bowl, combine the chicken, apples, cranberries, onion, and celery and mix well.

2.	In a small bowl, combine the mustard, mayonnaise, salt, and pepper and whisk together until well blended.

3.	Stir the dressing into the chicken mixture until thoroughly combined.

Savory Avocado Spread
Servings: 6

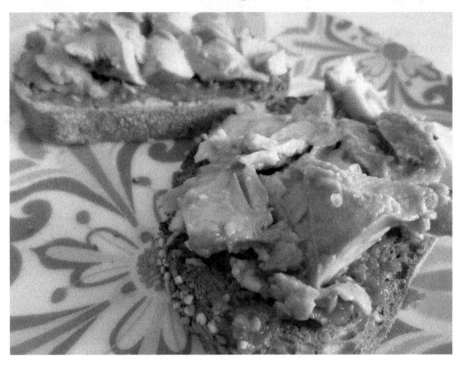

Ingredients

- 1 ripe avocado, peeled and pitted
- 1 teaspoon freshly squeezed lemon juice
- • 6 boneless sardine filets (packed in olive oil)
- 1/4 cup diced sweet white onion
- 1 stalk celery, diced
- 1/2 teaspoon salt
- 1/4 teaspoon freshly ground black pepper

Directions

1.   In a blender or food processor, combine the avocado, lemon juice, and sardine filets and pulse just until fairly smooth. A few chunks are fine for texture.

2.   Spoon the mixture into a small bowl and add the onion, celery, salt, and pepper. Mix well with a fork and serve as desired.

Barcelona baguette
Servings: 4

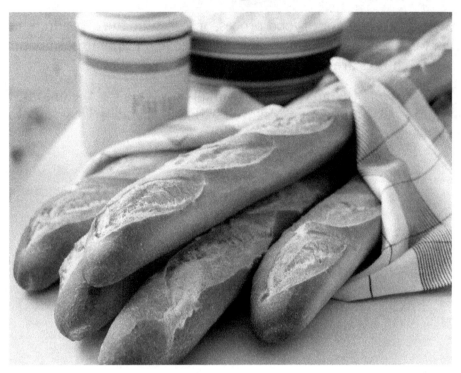

Ingredients:

- whole-wheat baguette
- 4 slices serrano ham, or similar large ripe tomatoes, halved
- 2-3 tablespoons olive oil
- Handful rocket leaves or arugula

Directions:

1.   In a lengthwise manner, split the baguette into halves. Drizzle the cut sides with the olive oil.

2.   Squeeze the pup of the tomato halves into the bread. Cover one baguette half with the ham and then scatter with the rocket leaves.

3.   Cover with the other baguette half; press down.

4.   Divide into 4 portions and tightly wrap each with foil.

Crispy Italian chicken with polenta
Servings: 2

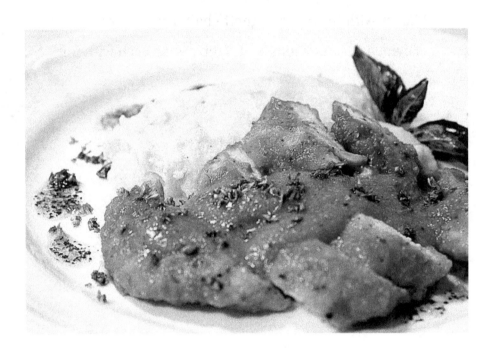

Ingredients:

- garlic clove, sliced
- fillets chicken breast, skin-on, boneless
- tablespoons olive oil
- 25 g Parmesan, grated
- 250 g pack cherry tomatoes,
- 500 g pack ready-to-use polenta
- Leaves from a few sprigs rosemary, torn

Directions:

1.   Preheat the oven to 220C, gas to7, or fan to 200C.

2.   With your fingers, roughly break the polenta into small chunks; scatter into the bottom of a small-sized roasting tin. Add the parmesan cheese; mix with the polenta.

3.   With the skin side up, place the chicken breast on top of the polenta mixture. Scatter the cherry tomatoes, the rosemary, and then the garlic over; drizzle with the olive oil and season to taste.

4.   Roast for about 25 minutes, until the chicken skin is golden and crispy and the cheese and the polenta are turning crusty around the edges.

5.   Serve with green salad.

Halloumi, Grape Tomato And Zucchini Skewers With Spinach-Basil Oil

Servings: 4

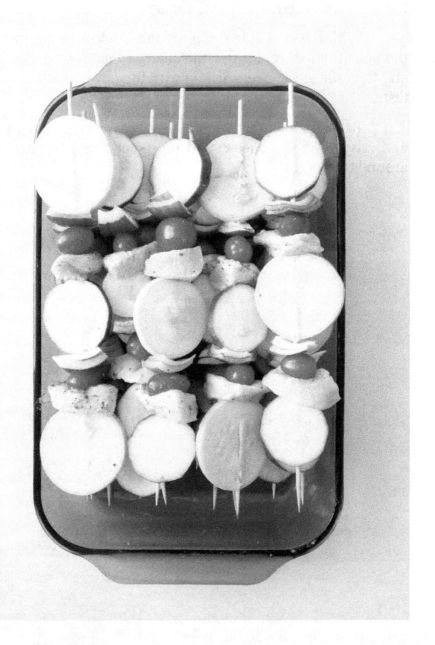

Ingredients:

- large zucchini, halved lengthways, cut into 8 pieces
- 16 grape tomatoes
- 180 g halloumi cheese, cut into 16 pieces
- Olive oil spray

For the spinach-basil oil:

- cups baby spinach leaves cups fresh basil leaves
- 185 ml (3/4 cup) extra-virgin olive oil
- 125 ml (1/2 cup) light olive oil

Directions:

1.   In a saucepan of boiling water, cook the spinach and the basil for about 30 seconds or until just wilted. Drain and cool under running cold water.

2.   Place the cooked spinach and basil into a food processor. Add the light olive oil and the extra-virgin olive oil; process until the mixture is smooth. Transfer into an airtight container, refrigerate for 8 hours to develop the flavors.

3.   Preheat the barbecue grill to medium-high.

4.   Thread a piece of zucchini, halloumi cheese, and tomato into each skewer. Lightly spray with the olive oil spray.

5.   Grill for about4 minutes per side or until cooked through and golden brown.

6. Arrange the grilled skewers on to serving platter; serve immediately with the prepared spinach-basil oil.

Balsamic Steak With Feta, Tomato, And Basil

Servings: 4

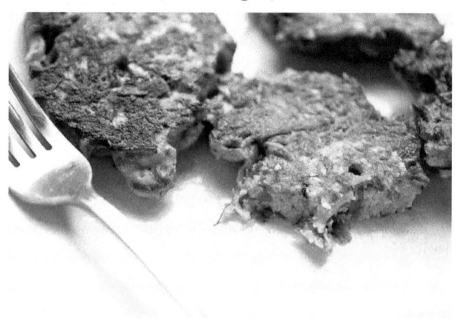

Ingredients:

- Tablespoon balsamic vinegar
- 1/4 cup basil leaves
- 175 g greek fetta, crumbled
- Tablespoons olive oil Teaspoons baby capers
- Sirloin steaks, trimmed
- Whole garlic cloves, skin on Roma tomatoes, halved
- Olive oil spray
- Salt and cracked black pepper

Directions:

1. Preheat the oven to 200C.

2. Line a baking tray with baking paper. Place the tomatoes and then scatter with the capers, crumbled feta, and the garlic cloves. Drizzle with 1 tablespoon of the olive oil and season with salt and pepper; cook for about 15 minutes or until the tomatoes are soft. Remove from the oven, set aside.

3. In a large non-metallic bowl, toss the steak with the remaining 1 tablespoon of olive oil, vinegar, salt and pepper; cover and refrigerate for 5 minutes.

4. Preheat the grill pan to high heat; grill the steaks for about 4 minutes per side or until cooked to your preference.

5. Serve with the prepared tomato mixture and sprinkle with basil.

Tomato, Roasted Peppers, And Feta Fritters

Servings: 12

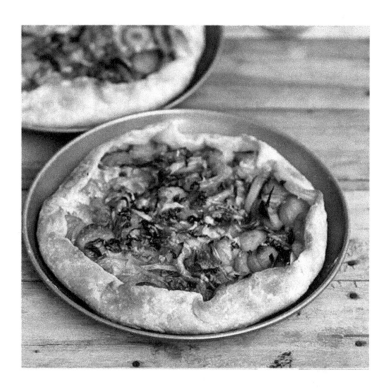

Ingredients:

- 1/2 cups self-rising whole-wheat flour
- Large tomato, deseeded, finely chopped
- 1/2 cup milk
- 1/3 cup (75 g) roasted peppers, finely chopped
- 1/4 cup canola oil
- Tablespoons parmesan cheese, finely grated (or vegetarian hard cheese)

- 200g feta, crumbled
- Eggs
- Pesto to serve

Directions:

1.   In a large mixing bowl, mix the eggs and the milk together.

2.   Place the flour in a large bowl, make a well in the center, and add the egg mixture; stir until the mixture is a smooth batter. Add the tomatoes, bell peppers, feta, and parmesan cheese.

3.   In a large-sized frying pan, heat 1 tablespoon oil over medium high heat. When the oil if add, pour 1 heaping tablespoon of the batter into the pan, flatten slightly. Repeat to make 7 fritters; cook for about 2-3 minutes per side or until cooked through and golden.

4.   Repeat the process to cook the remaining batter.

5.   Serve with nutty pesto.

Macedonian Greens And Cheese Pie
Servings: 6

Ingredients:

- Bunch chicory
- 1 bunch rocket or arugula 1 bunch mint
- 1 bunch dill
- 10 sheets whole-wheat filo pastry
- 150 g halloumi, finely diced
- 150 g ricotta
- 200 g baby spinach
- 250 g Greek feta, crumbled
- 4 eggs
- 50 g dried whole-wheat breadcrumbs
- 6 green onions, trimmed
- Olive oil, to brush

Directions:

1.   Trim the rocket stalks and the chicory. Finely chop the green onions and the dill (include the dill stems). Strip the mint leaves.

2.   Pour water into a large-sized pan; bring to boil. Ready a bowl with iced water beside the stove. Add the chicory into the boiling water; blanch for 3 minutes and using a slotted spoon, transfer to the bowl with iced water. Repeat the process with the spinach and the rocket, blanching each for 1 minute; drain well.

3.   A handful at a time, tightly wring the greens to squeeze out the excess liquid, then pat dry with paper towel. Finely chop the blanched greens. Combine them with the eggs, herbs, feta, 30 g of the breadcrumbs, ricotta, and 3/4 of the halloumi; season.

4.   Preheat the oven to 180C.

5.   Grease a 5.5-cm deep 25cmx pie tin.

6.   Brush a filo sheet with the olive oil, place it in the pie tin, extending the edge of the filo outside the edge of the tin. Brush the remaining sheets of filo and add them to the pie tin, arranging them like wheel spokes.

7.   Sprinkle the remaining breadcrumbs over the base of the layered filo sheets. Top with the filling mixture. Loosely fold the filo sheets over to cover the filling, brush with oil, sprinkle with water, and scatter the halloumi over.

8.   Bake for 45 minutes. After 45 minutes, cover, and bake for additional 15 minutes, or until heated through.

Mediterranean slices

Servings: 4

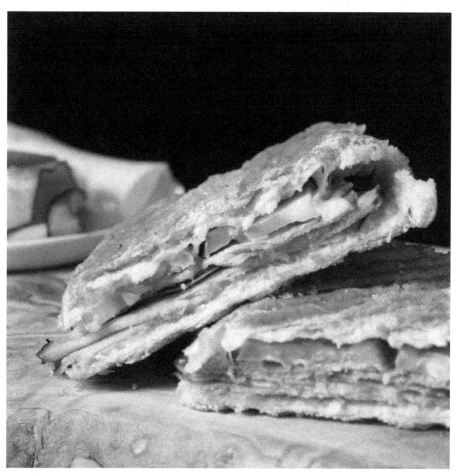

Ingredients:

125 g ball mozzarella, grated (or 85 g cheddar)

140 g roasted peppers, frozen, sliced

140g artichokes, frozen (about 3 wedges per serving)

375 g pack ready-rolled whole-wheat puff pastry

4 tablespoons green pesto

Directions

1.   Preheat the oven to 200C, gas to 6, or fan to 180C.

2.   Unroll the pastry and then cut into 4 rectangle pieces. With a sharp knife, cut a 1-cm edge inside each rectangle, making sure not to cut all the way through; place into a baking sheet.

3.   Into each slice, spread 1 tablespoon pesto, making sure to stay inside the border. Top with peppers and then with artichokes; bake for about 15 minutes until the pastry begins to brown.

4.   Scatter the grated mozzarella over the vegetables, return to the oven, and bake for additional 5 to 7 minutes, or until the cheese has melted and the pastry is crisp.

5.   Serve with green salad.

Mediterranean Tarts

Servings: 2

Ingredients:

Tablespoon pesto

1 teaspoon sugar, light muscovado

100 g Camembert cheese, cut into slices 100 g green bean, lightly steamed

Large onion, thinly sliced

Tablespoons olive oil, plus more

200 g cherry tomato on the vine, sliced into halves, reserve 2 sprigs with 3-4 tomatoes on each stem

Directions:

250 g ready-made whole-wheat puff pastry, thawed if frozen 50 g rocket leaves (arugula), preferably wild

6 anchovy fillets, optional 6 black olive, not pitted

6 medium new potato

A few basil leaves, roughly torn Good squeeze of lemon juice Knob butter

1.   Heat the butter with 1 tablespoon olive oil until the butter is melted. Add the onions; cook over medium-low heat for about

15-20 minutes, stirring often, until the onions are golden brown and soft.

2.   Add the sugar, stirring, and cook for 3 to 4 minutes more; remove from heat and let cool.

3.   Cook the potatoes in boiling salted water for about 10 minutes or until just tender; let cool enough to handle then slice.

4.   Preheat the oven to 220C, gas to 7, or fan to 200C.

5.   Divide the pastry into two; shape into rough rounds. On a lightly floured surface, roll each dough into 18-cm or 7-in rounds; place into baking sheet.

6.   Divide the caramelized onions between the two rounds, spreading to cove r the surface.

7.   Sprinkle the cheese over the onions. Top with the sliced potatoes, the sliced tomatoes, and if using, the anchovy fillets. Top with the reserved tomatoes on the vine. Scatter with the olives and drizzle with a bit of olive oil; bake for about 15 to 20 minutes, or until golden.

8.   Mix the pesto with the remaining 1 tablespoon of olive oil. Toss the beans and the rocket leaves with a little olive oil and the lemon juice; season.

9.   When the tarts are baked, drizzle the top with the pesto mixture.

10.   Serve with the green bean and rocket salad.

Mediterranean-Style Tuna Wrap

Servings: 4

Ingredients:

1/2 teaspoon lemon zest

1/4 cup fresh parsley, chopped 1/4 cup Kalamata olives, chopped 1/4 cup red onion, finely diced

2 cans (6-ounce each) chunk light tuna in water, drained well 2 large tomatoes, sliced

2 tablespoons lemon juice, freshly squeezed 3 tablespoons olive oil

4 whole-grain (about 2 ounces each) wrap breads 6 cups (about 3 ounces) mixed greens, pre-washed Freshly ground black pepper

Salt

Directions:

1.   In a medium mixing bowl, combine the tuna, parsley, onion, and olives.

2.   In a small mixing bowl, whisk the olive oil, lemon juice, lemon

zest, salt, and pepper. Pour about 2/3 of the dressing over the tuna mixture; toss to incorporate.

3.   In another bowl, combine the greens and the remaining 1/3 dressing; toss to coat.

4.   Into each piece of wrap bread, top tuna salad, then with 1 1/2 cup greens, and a few slices of tomatoes. Roll the wrap; serve.

Grilled Fish and Chunky Salsa with Avocado

Servings: 2

Ingredients:

Ripe avocado

Ripe plum tomato, each piece chopped into 6 chunks

1 small red onion, finely sliced

Tablespoons olive oil, plus more for drizzling Juice of 1/2 lemon or 1 lime

1   small bunch coriander, leaves only

2   pieces (140 g or 6 oz. Each) fish fillets, halibut or pacific cod, skin on

Directions:

1.   Halve and pit the avocado. Using a teaspoon, scoop out avocado chunks and put them in a large bowl.

2.   Except for fish fillets, gently mix the rest of the ingredients with the avocado chunks; set aside.

3.   Heat a griddle pan until very hot.

4.   Season the fillets with salt and pepper. If desired, drizzle with a bit of olive oil.

5.   When the griddle is hot, add the fish; cook for about 2-3 minutes per side, until cooked through and charred; serve with the chunky salsa.

Salami Ciabatta and Mozzarella

Servings: 2

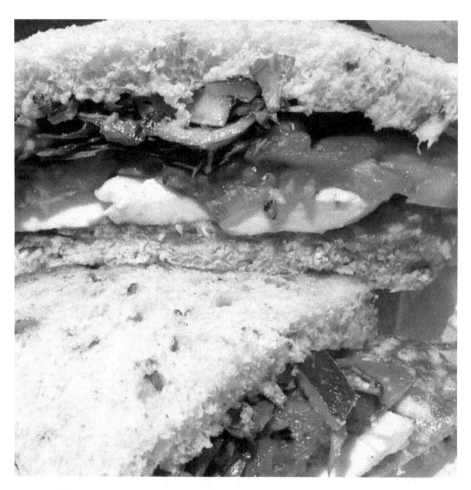

Ingredients:

1/2 of a 125 g ball mozzarella (if preferred, use a light version), drained, torn into pieces

handful rocket (arugula)

small fennel bulb, trimmed, thinly sliced

small whole-wheat ciabatta, split

1 tablespoon extra-virgin olive oil

8 slices salami, torn into pieces

Lemon wedges, for squeezing

Directions:

1. Cut the ciabatta into 4 slices; toast.

2. Toss the fennel and rocket/arugula with 2 teaspoons of the olive oil; season.

3. Rub the remaining olive oil over the cut sides of the ciabatta, then rub with garlic.

4. Divide the salami, mozzarella, and the fennel salad between the 4 bread slices, piling them; serve with the lemon wedges.

Baked Cheesy Spinach

Servings: 8

Ingredients:

bunch spring onions, finely sliced

6 sheets whole-wheat filo pastry

50 g Parmesan, grated

pieces (100 g-bag) baby spinach, chopped

200 g pack feta cheese

tablespoons olive oil

2 pieces (250 g each) tubs ricotta

100 g whole-wheat breadcrumbs egg

Nutmeg, grated

Directions:

1.   Heat the oven to 180C, gas to 4, or the fan to 160C.

2.   In a large-sized mixing bowl, mash the feta. Add the ricotta and then mash again until thoroughly mixed.

3.   Stir in the spring onions, spinach, egg, parmesan, nutmeg, 1/2 of the breadcrumbs, and season well.

4.   Lightly brush a 20x30-cm tin with olive oil.

5.   Layer 3 of the filo sheets into the tin, brushing each with olive oil before layering with the next sheet.

6.   Scatter the remaining 1/2 of the breadcrumbs over, evenly spreading. Spoon the ricotta over the breadcrumbs layer, spreading it gently to prevent dislodging the crumbs.

7.   Cover with the remaining filo, brushing with oil as you layer each piece. Cut into 6 to 8 portions and bake for about 35 to 40 minutes, or until the filo is crisp and golden; serve.

Beef and Wild Mushroom Stew

Servings: 8

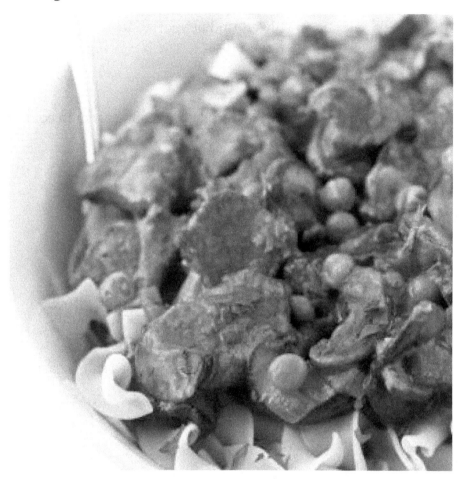

Ingredients

- 2 pounds fresh porcini or morel mushrooms

- 1/3 cup olive oil

- 2 pounds lean, boneless beef, cut into 2-inch cubes

- • 2 medium onions, finely chopped

- 1 clove garlic, minced

- 1 cup dry white wine

- 1 teaspoon thyme, minced

- • Sea salt and freshly ground pepper, to taste

Directions

1.   Wash the mushrooms carefully by soaking them in cold water and swirling them around.

2.   Trim away any soft parts of the mushrooms.

3.   Heat the olive oil over medium-high heat. Brown the meat evenly on all sides and set aside on a plate.

4.   Add the onions, garlic, and mushrooms to the olive oil, and cook for 5–8 minutes

5.   Cover and bring to a boil, then reduce heat to low and simmer. Simmer for 1 hour, or until the meat is tender and flavorful.

6.   Season with freshly ground pepper and sea salt to taste.

Chicken and Potato Tagine

Servings: 6

Ingredients

- 1 chicken, cut up into 8 pieces
- 1 medium onion, thinly sliced
- 3 cloves garlic, minced
- 1/4 cup olive oil
- 1/2 teaspoon ground cumin
- 1/2 teaspoon freshly ground pepper
- 1/4 teaspoon ginger
- • Pinch saffron threads
- 1 teaspoon paprika
- Sea salt, to taste

- 2 cups water
- 3 cups potatoes, peeled and diced
- 1/2 cup flat-leaf parsley, chopped
- 1/2 cup fresh cilantro, chopped
- • 1 cup fresh or frozen green peas

Directions

1.   Place the chicken, onion, garlic, olive oil, and seasonings into a Dutch oven. Add about 2 cups water and bring to a boil

over medium-high heat. Reduce heat and cover. Simmer for 30 minutes.

2.   Add the potatoes, parsley, and cilantro, and simmer an additional 20 minutes, or until the potatoes are almost tender.

3.   Add the peas at the last moment, simmering for an additional 5 minutes. Serve hot.

Lebanese Grilled Chicken

Servings: 4

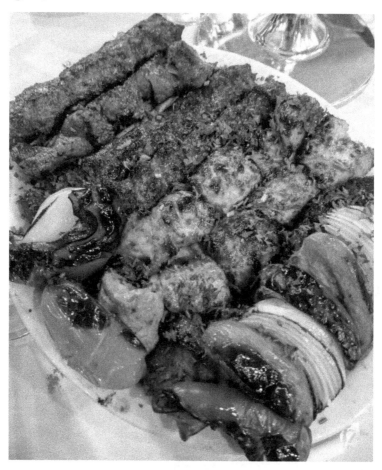

Ingredients

- 1/2 cup olive oil

- 1/4 cup apple cider vinegar

- Zest and juice of 1 lemon

- 4 cloves garlic, minced

- • 2 teaspoons sea salt

- 1 teaspoon Arabic 7 spices (baharaat)

- 1/2 teaspoon cinnamon

- • 1 chicken, cut into 8 pieces

Directions

1.   Combine all the ingredients except the chicken in a shallow dish or plastic bag.

2.   Place the chicken in the bag or dish and marinate overnight, or at least for several hours.

3.   Drain, reserving the marinade. Heat the grill to medium-high.

4.   Cook the chicken pieces for 10–14 minutes, brushing them with the marinade every 5 minutes or so.

5.   The chicken is done when the crust is golden brown and an instant-read thermometer reads 180 degrees in the thickest parts. Remove skin before eating.

Arroz con Pollo

Servings: 6

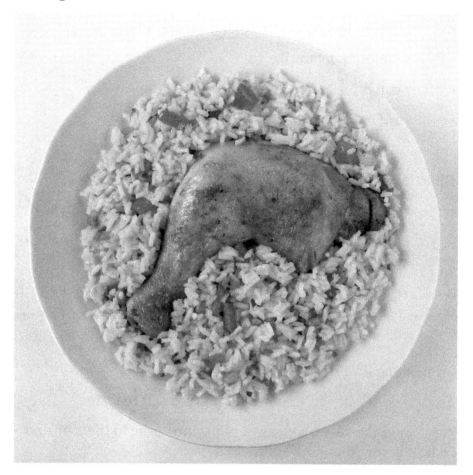

Ingredients:

- 4 tablespoons olive oil
- 1 chicken, cut into pieces
- Sea salt and freshly ground pepper, to taste
- 3 sweet red peppers, coarsely chopped
- 1 onion, chopped

- • 2 garlic cloves, minced
- 2 1/2 cups chicken stock
- 1 (14-ounce) can diced tomatoes, drained
- 1 tablespoon paprika
- 1 cup brown rice
- • 1/4 cup flat-leaf parsley, chopped

Directions

1. Heat the olive oil in a large skillet on medium-high heat.

2. Place the chicken in the pan, and cook it 8–10 minutes, or until lightly browned on both sides.

3. Transfer the chicken to an oven-safe dish, and keep warm in the

oven on the lowest setting.

4. Add freshly ground pepper and sea salt to taste.

5. Add the sweet peppers, onion, and garlic to the pan, and cook, stirring frequently, until tender.

6. Heat the chicken stock in the microwave or a saucepan until simmering. Add the chicken stock, tomatoes, and paprika to the pan.

7. Stir in the rice, and place the chicken pieces on top.

8. Simmer with the lid on for 20–30 minutes, or until the liquid is absorbed and the rice is tender.

9. Garnish with parsley.

10. Serve with a green salad or tomato and red

onion salad.

Greek Kebabs

Servings: 6

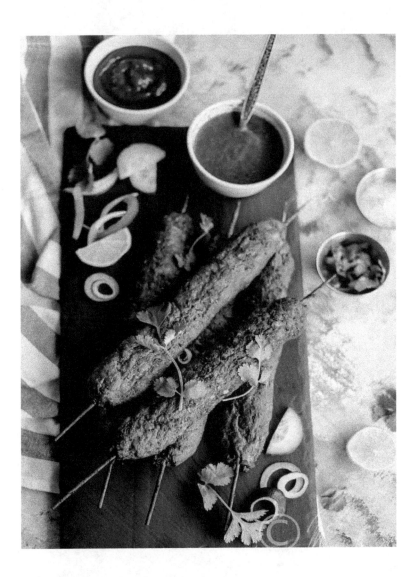

- 1/4 cup olive oil
- Juice of 1 lemon

- 1 tablespoon dried oregano

- 2 cloves garlic, minced

- • 5 bay leaves

- Sea salt and freshly ground pepper, to taste

- • 2 pounds beef sirloin, cut into 2-inch cubes

Directions

1.   Combine all the ingredients except the meat in a plastic bag. Add the meat and shake to coat.

2.   Marinate for up to 24 hours and drain.

3.   Skewer the meat onto 8-inch skewers and grill on medium heat for 8–10 minutes, turning the skewers halfway through the cooking time.

CPSIA information can be obtained
at www.ICGtesting.com
Printed in the USA
LVHW081110210321
681561LV00049B/137